# Dr. on Cancer, Weight Loss, Alternative Medicine and More

Dr. Aleathea R. Wiggins

## Disclaimer

This book is a collection of health articles based on the Dr. Oz show. It is designed to provide general information about a number of common medical conditions and tips for healthy living. It is not intended to be a substitute for consulting with your physician or receiving appropriate medical treatment. The author shall have neither liability nor responsibility to any person or entity with respect to any loss or damage caused, or alleged to have been caused, directly or indirectly, by the information contained in this book.

Copyright © 2014 Aleathea R. Wiggins

All rights reserved.

**ISBN-13**: 978-1495980497
**ISBN-10**: 1495980499

*For Chaelin,*
*You are my everything.*

# Contents

Introduction .................................................................... 7

## Part 1 - Dr. Oz on Cancer
Water and Cancer ............................................................ 9
Pancreatic Cancer ........................................................... 11
Radiation ........................................................................ 12
Thyroid Guards ............................................................... 15
5 Causes of Cancer ......................................................... 17
Oral Cancer .................................................................... 19
Esophageal Cancer ......................................................... 20
Stomach Cancer ............................................................. 21
Breast Cancer Prevention ................................................ 22
Cancer-Fighting Food ...................................................... 24
Anti-Cancer Spices ......................................................... 26
Antioxidants and Cancer .................................................. 27

## Part 2 - Dr. Oz on Weight Loss
Practical Weight Loss Tips ............................................... 29
Eat to Lose Weight .......................................................... 32
10 Commandments for Weight Loss .................................. 33
Fat Busters ..................................................................... 35
Burn Fat to Lose Weight ................................................... 37
The Best Frozen Food to Lose Weight ............................... 38
Think Yourself Skinny ...................................................... 39
Lap Band Surgery ........................................................... 41

## Part 3 - Dr. Oz on Alternative Medicine
Alternative Medicine.................................................. 45
Acupuncture............................................................ 47
Acupuncture for Cancer............................................ 48
Alternative Treatments for Pain................................. 50
Medical Marijuana.................................................... 51
The Hero of Alternative Medicine.............................. 55

## Part 4 - Dr. Oz on Anti-Aging
Anti-Aging Tips........................................................ 58
Botox Considerations............................................... 60
Look Younger.......................................................... 61
HGH - Human Growth Hormone................................ 62

## Part 5 - Dr. Oz on Healthy Living
Boost Your Immune System...................................... 64
Super Charge Your Health........................................ 66
Take Vitamins.......................................................... 67
7 Day Energy Surge................................................. 68
How to Stop Smoking............................................... 70
The Weekend Challenge.......................................... 71
Live to Be 100......................................................... 73

## Part 6 - Dr. Oz on Medical Conditions
Chronic Fatigue Syndrome....................................... 76
Hysterectomy and Fibroids...................................... 78
Preventing Alzheimer's............................................ 80
Sciatica................................................................... 82
Women's Depression............................................... 83
Heart Attack............................................................ 85
Heart Attack Warning Signs..................................... 87
Heartburn................................................................ 88

## Part 7 - Dr. Oz on Food and Drinks
Organic Food is Better............................................... 91
Herbal Tea............................................................ 93
Immunity Boosting Food........................................... 95
Dr. Oz on Soda....................................................... 96
Food for Memory..................................................... 97
Spices for Health..................................................... 99

Conclusion..............................................................102

*Acknowledgments......................................................103*
*About the Author.....................................................104*

# Introduction

**Reasons We Love and Trust Dr. Oz**

Why do so many people love Dr. Oz? Is it because he is intelligent and down-to-earth with a great sense of humor? Is it because he is not afraid of admitting that doctors are not God, and they need to get over their God complexes? Whatever the reason, Dr. Oz sure does have a lot of fans. Men and women around the world tune in daily to the Dr. Oz show.

These days there is a lot of controversy in the world of medicine and doctors are losing trust among patients. It is refreshing that Dr. Oz is able to maintain a high level of trust. Thousand of people around the world respect his medical opinions and appreciate his open-mindedness. Dr. Oz believes in giving the people a voice. He encourages patients to ask questions and to be assertive when necessary in order to get their health needs addressed. This is one of the main reasons so many people love him and continue to offer their support.

Dr. Oz is not afraid to admit that he makes mistakes

or that he doesn't have all the answers. He is not concerned about causing a controversy or speaking out against popular views in the world of medicine. He is not worried about putting his peers on the spot on national television by making them answer the tough questions. He is not afraid to tell other doctors that they are wrong. He is a doctor for the people.

Of course, there are some folks who are not fans of the great Dr. Oz. There are people who absolutely hate him. And there are those who are involved in a love-hate relationship with the man. Never-the-less, we need more doctors like him practicing medicine because he is willing to look for answers. He is seeking the cause of diseases and honestly hoping for a cure, while too many doctors are going through the motions just treating symptoms.

Although I do not always agree with his perspective, I will remain a Dr. Oz fan because I believe that he sincerely wants to make people healthier and help improve their quality of life. Tune in to Dr. Oz. You will laugh a lot and learn even more and it might just save your life.

# Part 1
# Dr. Oz on Cancer

### **Water and Cancer**

Dr. Oz shared the unfortunate truth that your drinking water could be causing cancer. Tap water often contains unsafe levels of toxic chemicals which could lead to cancer and other serious health problems, such as kidney disease, liver damage and tumors in the mouth.

The only way to determine if your water is safe is to test it for toxic chemicals. According to Dr. Oz, it is important to look out for chromium-6, lead, arsenic and perchlorate. These are cancer causing chemicals that will wreak havoc on your health. Presently, the government does not appear to be doing enough to keep drinking water safe. Dr. Oz took water samples from around the country to test. He found that some of the water that families were drinking every day contained harmful chemicals.

"Many of the health problems that we are seeing

today that are blamed on environmental factors are actually a result of the water we are drinking," said Dr. Oz. "Toxins in the water can cause memory problems and even raise your blood pressure," warned Dr. Oz. Toxins in the water may also be linked to thyroid problems.

There are certain areas across the country with unexplainable high levels of cancer rates, especially leukemia among children. This could be a direct result of toxic water. Although the EPA is taking some steps to help make tap water safer, there are steps that everyone should take to protect their health.

Dr. Oz recommends checking the Consumer Confidence Report for your area to find out about the quality of your tap water. In some cities it may be possible to get a free water test kit from the health department. Dr. Oz also stressed the importance of getting educated about the health risks associated with toxic water. In the meantime, use a water filter.

Are you drinking cancer causing water? If you find your water to be toxic get involved and demand improvements in your city. Also, be sure to share this information with your health care provider. It might explain

## Pancreatic Cancer

Pancreatic cancer is the most feared of all types of cancer because it is the deadliest, according to Dr. Oz. Pancreatic cancer is extremely serious because by the time it is discovered it has already spread out in the body and it may be too late to effectively treat it.

Pancreatic cancer is very difficult to detect in the early stages because there are simply no effective screening methods for this type of cancer. However, it is possible to lower your risks for pancreatic cancer by changing your diet. One step is to reduce the amount of fatty red meat in your diet while increasing your intake of colorful vegetables and fruits, which contain high levels of anti-cancer properties.

Two of the most common symptoms of pancreatic cancer are stomach pain and backaches. Additional warning signs that Dr. Oz explained include pale colored stools, jaundice and dark colored urine. People who are experiencing these symptoms should be evaluated by a medical doctor as soon as possible.

"Pancreatic cancer scares me," admitted Dr. Oz.

Pancreatic cancer can grow and spread in the body for decades before it is diagnosed. The pancreas is hidden behind other organs which makes it more problematic for doctors to screen.

There is a lot of research focused on pancreatic cancer and a new vaccine has been developed which may help in the fight against the disease. Currently, doctors are trying to develop a blood test to detect early stages of pancreatic cancer.

**Radiation**

"The Dr. Oz show controversy: The Radiation Risk Your Doctor Doesn't Think is Real" sparked a heated debate. Dr. Oz urges the public to request thyroid guards when getting dental x-rays and mammograms.

According to Dr. Oz, it is essential to take appropriate steps to protect yourself from unnecessary exposure to radiation. Currently, thyroid cancer is the fastest growing cancer in women and this could be the result of radiation exposure. "Ask for a lead thyroid guard to protect your thyroid when you get a dental x-ray," warned Dr. Oz.

Most dental offices do not have thyroid guards on

hand and some of the offices that do have the guards fail to offer them to the patients for use. However, research has demonstrated that "people who received more than 5 dental x-rays in a lifetime have more than 5 times the rate of developing thyroid cancer," stated Dr. Oz.

Thyroids guards cost about $25.00 and should be available at all dental offices for extra protection against radiation exposure. One dental hygienist on the Dr. Oz show stated that she became very concerned about the safety of her patients so she ordered the thyroid shields to help protect against radiation.

However, some doctors who appeared on the Dr. Oz show think that thyroid guards are unnecessary, stating that "the amount of radiation exposure from dental x-rays and mammograms is very small." Dr. Oz insists that it makes sense to wear the shield to reduce the level of exposure ." Why not take the extra precaution? Isn't it better to make radiation exposure even smaller? We do not know the long-term effects of the radiation exposure. Who knows what those results will be 10 years from now."

In fact, Dr. Oz pointed out that both the ADA and government have concerns about radiation. "The American

Dental Association and the U.S. government now recommend using the thyroid guard when getting x-rays. So why not use the protection?" questioned Dr. Oz. "Even with mammography use the thyroid guard. Take any precaution you can to protect the precious thyroid tissue," he added.

Dr. Oz explained that x-ray technicians always leave the room or use x-ray shields to protect themselves because they have concerns. "It is also important to understand the patients' concerns," he said. "I wear a shield when I'm working in the hospital to protect myself from radiation," admitted Dr. Oz.

Dr. Oz acknowledged that he understands the controversy and that some doctors may not agree with him. However, he stands firm on his professional, medical opinion. "These are my final recommendations about the thyroid guard. With dental x-rays, wear it. Mammograms, ask for a thyroid guard shield," insisted Dr. Oz.

"One of the problems with doctors is that we don't always hear the patients, but I believe patients have a right to control their care." said Dr. Oz.

## **Thyroid Guards**

Wearing a thyroid guard during mammograms and dental x-rays may help protect you against thyroid cancer, which happens to be the fastest growing cancer among women. In addition, the rate of thyroid cancer in men is increasing.

Patients should request the use of a thyroid guard during x-ray procedures. Dr. Oz, warned that repeated mammograms and dental x-rays contribute to the development of thyroid cancer and recommends the use of thyroid guards. Likewise, the American Dental Association recommends wearing thyroid guards during x-rays to reduce radiation exposure.

However, there is some concern among doctors that thyroid guards could obscure the view of mammograms in some patients. Patients and doctors will need to discuss this concern on an individual basis. In most cases thyroid guards do not affect mammogram screenings.

Minimizing radiation exposure is important for the prevention of cancer. It is a documented fact that radiation is cumulative and exposure is a risk factor for thyroid cancer.

A large number of dental and medical offices do not have thyroid shields. Call in advance before scheduling an appointment to make sure thyroid guards are available. Ask for a thyroid guard during the appointment if the medical staff fails to offer you one. Do not worry about offending anyone. Protecting your health by limiting exposure to radiation is the priority.

With the health care crisis in America at an all time high, more people are focusing on preventive care. Thyroid guards are one preventive measure against thyroid cancer and cost as little as $25 each. Health care professionals should have them available for their patients. Reducing radiation exposure even in small doses is beneficial to overall health.

There are other steps you can take to help prevent thyroid cancer and other cancers as well. It is essential to take personal responsibility for your health. This means weighing the benefits and risks of all medical procedures and drugs. Do the research, ask questions and get multiple medical opinions. Do not be afraid to speak up if you do not agree with your doctor's advice. It is your body and doctors make mistakes all the time. You have a right to control the kind of care you receive.

## **5 Causes of Cancer**

Dr. Oz explained 5 causes of cancer that can be controlled. "People can greatly reduce the risks of cancer by making these simple lifestyle changes," said Dr. Oz.

***Vitamin E and Cancer.*** "Getting too much vitamin E could cause lung cancer," said Dr. Oz. In general, vitamin E is beneficial because it contains useful antioxidants which help protect the body. However, in extremely high doses, vitamin E damages DNA and contributes to the development of cancer. Dr. Oz recommends getting vitamin E naturally through the diet instead of taking supplements. Nuts, such as pistachios, are high in vitamin E.

***Inconsistent Mealtimes and Cancer.*** Another possible cause of cancer is the lack of routine meal times. It is better for the body to eat meals on a fixed schedule. Eat breakfast, lunch and dinner at approximately the same time each day. "Eating at different times causes stress in the body, which leads to insulin spikes and inflammation throughout the body that causes cancer," explained Dr. Oz.

***Poor Dental Care and Cancer.*** Failing to take care of your teeth can cause cancer. According to Dr. Oz, plaque buildup on the teeth causes inflammation that travels through the body which can eventually lead to cancer anywhere in the body. Several studies show a link between various forms of cancer and poor oral hygiene. Thus, carefully brushing and flossing your teeth daily are important steps in cancer prevention.

***Lack of Sleep and Cancer.*** Research has verified a link between sleep deprivation and cancer. Sleep deprivation increases the risk of developing polyps in the colon. Additionally, our bodies produce melatonin, which helps repair cells during periods of sleep. Damaged cells that are not repaired could cause cancer. "Adults really should sleep between 7 and 8 hours each night," advised Dr. Oz.

***Low Fat Diet Foods and Cancer.*** Dr. Oz explained how low-fat diet foods cause cancer. "These foods overload the body with simple carbohydrates and fillers which cause damage to the body. They cause your insulin to spike and again this leads to inflammation which can cause cancer," warned Dr. Oz. Moreover, low-fat diet foods lead to increased food cravings causing you to eat more while failing to provide your body with the protective fat that it needs.

## **Oral Cancer**

Oral cancer kills one person every hour, according to Dr. Oz, and is linked to the HPV or Human Papilloma Virus. Dr. Oz urges everyone to get screened for oral cancer and to be aware of the warning signs of the disease.

"Oral cancer is easy to diagnose and treat, but most cases are found too late," explained Dr. Oz. If found early, most cases of oral cancer are curable. In the past, oral cancer was a disease that affected mostly men. People that smoked or drank alcohol were at a higher risk. Recently, most new cases of oral cancer are attributed to the HPV.

Dr. Oz listed the following warning signs and symptoms of oral cancer. Seek immediate medical assistance if you recognize any of these signs in yourself.

***White or Red Patches in the Mouth.*** "If you have white or red patches in your mouth or sores that will not heal, this is cause for concern," explained Dr. Oz.

***Ear Pain or Sore Throat.*** Ear pain associated with oral cancer is generally experienced on one side and in one ear. An unexplained sore throat in the absence of a cold or flu may be an indication of oral cancer.

***A Lump in the Neck.*** According to Dr. Oz, this sign of oral cancer usually occurs at the advanced stages after the cancer has spread from your tongue and lymph nodes into your neck.

***Voice Changes or Hoarseness.*** Dr. Oz recommends getting checked for oral cancer if you experience this symptom for more than a week. It is possible to have tumors growing around your vocal chords.

## Esophageal Cancer

"You may already have esophageal cancer without knowing it," warned Dr. Oz, who claims that esophageal cancer is now the fastest growing cancer in America. According to Dr. Oz, risk factors for esophageal cancer include a high acid diet. Foods high in acid or those that contribute to acid production in the stomach include chocolate, alcohol, coffee, breath mints, raw tomatoes and raw garlic. Another big risk factor for esophageal cancer is smoking cigarettes. Dr. Oz advises people to give up smoking and to avoid eating high acid foods. He also recommends not eating within 3 hours of your bedtime.

Dr. Oz stresses the importance of paying attention to warning signs. "Reflux can be an early sign of esophageal cancer," said Dr. Oz. Additional symptoms include persistent hoarseness or sore throats, persistent cough, a lump in the throat and post-nasal drip. Difficulty or pain swallowing, unexplained weight loss and frequent heartburn are also indications that you could have esophageal cancer.

If you are experiencing these symptoms get checked by a doctor as soon as possible. Prolonging a check-up if you have cancer will allow the cancer time to progress further. Early detection is often your best defense.

## **Stomach Cancer**

"Stomach cancer is currently on the rise among Caucasian women," said Dr. Oz. "Generally, stomach cancer was high among African-Americans and Latinos." It is important to know the signs of stomach cancer and to be assertive in seeking treatment because stomach cancer is sometimes misdiagnosed as stress.

***Signs of Stomach Cancer.*** According to Dr. Oz,

symptoms of stomach cancer usually include abdominal pain and discomfort. In the beginning stages people experience nausea, which then progresses to vomiting. Lack of appetite and weight loss are also common signs that you may have stomach cancer.

***Causes of Stomach Cancer.*** Some cases of stomach cancer are attributed to the H. Pylori bacteria, which infects the stomach and often causes peptic ulcers. "About half of the population is infected with this bacteria, but it does not affect everyone in the same way," advised Dr. Oz.

Another contributing factor for developing stomach cancer is diet. "When I was in medical school I always associated stomach cancer with old men who smoked and drank. Now I know stomach cancer can affect anyone. You can reduce your chances of developing stomach cancer by eating certain foods and avoiding others," said Dr. Oz. Processed and smoked meats, like hot dogs, may contribute to stomach cancer because they are high in nitrates and nitrites, so limit your intake of these types of meats.

## Breast Cancer Prevention

Breast cancer is a leading cause of death among

women. Following the advice of Dr. Oz may help reduce your risks of developing breast cancer.

**Consume Breast Cancer Fighting Foods.** Dr. Oz recommends using food as medicine for the prevention of breast cancer. Certain foods, such as green tea are high in antioxidants which help strengthen the immune system. Green tea not only helps build immunity, but is also helps your body destroy cancer cells. According to Dr. Oz, drinking 3 cups of green tea daily could help reduce your chances of getting breast cancer by 50%. Garlic, leafy green vegetables and olive oil are also at the top of Dr. Oz's cancer fighting food list.

**Get Vitamin D Daily.** Vitamin D is believed to help prevent breast cancer. Thus, Dr. Oz recommends getting vitamin D everyday, even if that means taking a supplement. Many foods are fortified with vitamin D, but one of the best ways to get vitamin D is to spend 15 minutes a day soaking in the sun.

**Take Aspirin.** According to Dr. Oz, taking aspirin twice a week will help cut your chances of developing breast cancer by as much as 28%. Several studies, including a study published in the *Journal of the National Cancer Institute*, indicate that taking aspirin helps prevent and reduce recurrence of breast cancer.

## **Cancer-Fighting Foods**

Cancer fighting foods are cheap and readily available. Dr. Oz discussed ways to reduce cancer risks by making small dietary changes. Currently, there is no known cure for cancer. Taking steps to prevent cancer may be more practical than waiting for a cure. There are many foods that help prevent the development of cancer. Three of the best choices of cancer fighting foods were presented on the Dr. Oz show.

*Wild Blueberries.* Wild blueberries are a known super food rich in antioxidants, which help protect the body from free radicals. Although all blueberries offer health benefits, wild blueberries are the most effective for fighting cancer. Mary Ann Lila, PhD, a guest on the Dr. Oz show, conducted several studies related to the health benefits of wild blueberries. Her studies indicated that "the compounds in wild blueberries may be effective inhibitors of both the initiation and promotion stages of cancer," (*Journal of Agricultural and Food Chemistry, 2004*). Wild blueberries can be purchased in the frozen foods section of most supermarkets.

**Black Currants.** Black currants are an excellent cancer fighting food. They are a great source of vitamins, nutrients, antioxidants and other compounds which help protect against breast cancer, colon cancer and other diseases. Black currants are also known to enhance the effectiveness of cancer treatments. Black currants can be purchased at health food stores and many grocery stores in the form of juice and jam. They are also available in a dried form, similar to raisins, and as a tea.

**Muscadine Grapes.** Muscadine grapes are one of the best sources of polyphenolic antioxidants and other cancer fighting substances. Studies using muscadine grape components have indicated health benefits in the fight against blood cancer, colon cancer and prostate cancer. Muscadine grapes can be eaten fresh or consumed in the form of wine, juice and jelly. Muscadine grape products are available at most health stores.

Additional cancer fighting foods include tomatoes, spinach, broccoli, onions and garlic. These fruits and vegetables are high in vitamins and nutrients, and they contain properties that help detoxify the body.

Reduce your chances of developing cancer by

including cancer fighting foods in your daily diet. "Small things done everyday make a difference. This is how we're going to beat cancer," said Dr. Oz.

## **Anti-Cancer Spices**

You can reduce your chances of developing cancer while enriching the flavor of your favorite foods with anti-cancer spices. Dr. Oz recommends mixing together thyme, rosemary, peppermint, spearmint and sage. Keep the mixture in a small shaker to make it convenient to sprinkle on your lunch and dinner each day.

***Thyme***. Thyme is a leading spice for supporting good health. Not only is thyme rich in cancer-fighting antioxidants, it also contains iron, calcium and vitamin K.

***Rosemary***. Used medicinally throughout history, rosemary continues to be a popular anti-cancer spice. Other benefits include pain relief and memory improvement.

***Peppermint***. Peppermint is one of the healthiest anti-cancer spices around. According to preliminary studies, peppermint oil components may be able to kill cancer cells without damaging to healthy cells.

***Spearmint.*** Essential oil and stem components from

the spearmint tree are commonly used to prepare cancer remedies for natural health. Spearmint is also beneficial for depression and digestive problems.

***Sage.*** Sage is another beneficial spice that contains anti-cancer properties. In addition to sprinkling sage on your favorite meals, you might enjoy drinking sage tea.

## **Antioxidants and Cancer**

Too much of a good thing can be harmful to your health. According to Dr. Oz, taking too many antioxidant supplements is a dangerous practice because it actually increases your chances of getting cancer. Dr. Oz shared this information after a new study came out that revealed the problems with antioxidant supplements.

"It is best to get antioxidants from food sources. Those do not raise your risk of developing cancer. But, we need to be careful when it comes to supplements, " advised Dr. Oz. A healthy diet, which consists of a variety of plant-based foods, will help you get the antioxidants you need.

Dr. Oz recommends eating a colorful diet. Green,blue, red, yellow, orange and purple fruits and vegetables are rich in essential vitamins and minerals. So, try to eat more blueberries, cherries, collard greens and other brightly colored produce.

Antioxidants are good for you when they come from natural food sources. Those will help you ward off cancer and other illnesses. If your body is lacking in proper nutrients consult your health care provider or a registered dietitian. Stocking up on antioxidant supplements and other vitamins is not the solution for a poor diet.

# Part 2

# Dr. Oz on Weight Loss

## Practical Weight Loss Tips

"The incidence of heart disease, diabetes and arthritis can be cut in half just by losing 10 pounds," explained Dr. Oz. Even if you are 50 pounds overweight setting a primary goal to lose 10 pounds will make a huge difference in your health.

Dr. Oz advises dieters to start out small on their weight loss journey. Make basic lifestyle changes and watch those pounds begin to shed. Here are a few tried and true weight loss tips from Dr. Oz.

***Eat Breakfast.*** According to Dr. Oz, eating a fiber-rich breakfast, such as oatmeal, is essential for successful weight loss. Fiber-rich meals help control hunger and keep blood sugar stable.

***Eat an Apple and Walnuts.*** Dr. Oz recommends

eating an apple and walnuts before meals. Apples are extremely nutritious and they will satisfy your appetite. Walnuts are known as brain food because they keep you alert and energized. If you eat an apple and walnuts before lunch or dinner, you're more likely to eat less during your meal, which will help you lose weight.

***Dilute Juice.*** Mixing water into your juice will help you cut down on calories. You will definitely be getting less sugar. As an added benefit you will increase your water intake. Do not worry about losing vitamins from diluting your juice. Instead, eat plenty of fruits.

***Use Applesauce Instead of Oil.*** Another great weight loss tip from Dr. Oz is to substitute applesauce in baking recipes that call for vegetable oil. The dish will taste the same, but the fat content will be minimized. Next time you bake a cake or cornbread forget the oil and use applesauce.

***Stop Drinking Soda.*** According to Dr. Oz, replacing just one can of soda a day with a glass of water will make a significant difference in your ability to successfully lose weight. Soda is simply a can full of sugar or high fructose corn syrup. Even diet soda can impede your weight loss efforts because the artificial sweeteners found in diet soda may increase your appetite and cause food cravings.

***Add Cayenne Pepper.*** Not only will adding cayenne pepper enhance the flavor of your food, but it could help you lose weight. According to Dr. Oz, "Cayenne pepper has been proven to burn fat."

***Take a Walk.*** Even short periods of moderate exercise will support your weight loss efforts. Dr. Oz recommends getting at least 10 minutes of physical exercise each day. This can be accomplished by taking a daily walk. If you are short on time, take walks during your lunch break.

***Use Portion Control.*** "Do not eat snack portions larger than the size of your fist," advises Dr. Oz. Sometimes how much you eat is just as important as what you eat. You can automatically reduce your food serving sizes and lose weight by using smaller plates and having only one serving. If the meal doesn't fill you up, drink a glass of water.

When it comes to weight loss, small steps lead to big improvements. Follow the tips of Dr. Oz as you begin your journey towards losing weight the healthy way.

## **Eat to Lose Weight**

If you want to lose weight you've got to eat. Starvation diets do not work. Being hungry does not work. You have to eat in order to keep hunger under control so that you don't overeat.

When you eat to lose weight you need to know exactly what you are eating. Dr. Oz urges consumers to read food labels and pay close attention to the ingredients. Avoid all foods that list "simple sugars, bleached flour, high fructose corn syrup, saturated fat and trans fat" in the first five ingredients on the list.

Another great way to eat to lose weight is to eat at home and use smaller plates. According to Dr. Oz, "Small plates will change your life." When people use small plates they automatically eat less food. Stay away from large plates, large containers, or bags. Fix your meals and snacks on small plates and drink water before or during the meal.

Did you know that many people fail to lose weight because they confuse being thirty with being hungry? Don't make this mistake. Whenever you feel hungry drink a glass of water first because that might do the trick. Remember to drink at least eight glasses of water each day.

## Dr Oz's "10 Commandments for Weight Loss"

***1. Thou Shalt Not Wear Pants that Stretch.*** If your clothes grow with your body you won't notice the weight coming on making it more difficult to lose weight. Buy clothes that fit that are not made using stretchy material or elastic waistbands.

***2. Thou Shalt Not Keep Bad Clothes in Your Closet.*** As you lose weight trade in those big, baggy clothes for slim fitting wear. You'll be more likely to stay on track with healthy eating habits.

***3. Thou Shalt Not Eat Meat That Walks on Four Legs More Than Once a Week.*** Beef and pork should be eaten in moderation. Anything more leads to heart disease, increased cancer risks and obesity.

***4. Thou Shalt Not Graze in Search of Prey.*** Forget about window shopping in the refrigerator. Open it only to get what you need for pre-planned meals so you won't eat on impulse.

***5. Thou Shalt Not Eat After 7:30pm.*** Eating at night means eating larger amounts of junk foods, especially if you're watching television.

***6. Thou Shalt Not Pile Food More than One Inch High or Within Two Inches of the Plate Edge.*** Practice portion control. Try getting smaller plates and you will naturally eat less.

***7. Thou Shalt Not Chew Food Less than 20 Times Per Bite.*** Chewing allows your body to realize that you are eating food and to alert you when your stomach is full. Not chewing enough interferes with this process causing you to overeat.

***8. Thou Shalt Not Covet Thy Neighbor's Plate.*** Don't nibble off other peoples meals or snacks. Learn to say 'No thank you' when offered food. Otherwise, you could mindlessly add 1000 calories or more to your daily diet.

***9. Thou Shalt Not Carry Small Bills***. Small bills end up in vending machines while candy, chips and soda end up in your stomach.

### 10. Thou Shalt Not Eat While Standing Up.

When you stand you are more likely to eat faster and to consume more. Sitting down will help you eat slower and focus on how much you are eating.

## Fat Busters

"Replacing one meal a day is all it takes to control your body's fat," announced Dr. Oz as he shared fat busters that conquer problem areas of the body. According to Dr. Oz, it is possible to alter your body chemistry with the food you eat.

***Big Bottom.*** Having a big behind is a common complaint of many women. Dr. Oz's fat buster for big butts is the red clover meal. The meal consists of drinking 2 cups of red clover tea and dining on pasta primavera. For best results it is necessary to consume this fat buster in place of one meal everyday for five days.

***Big Belly.*** "Fat on the belly is the most dangerous," said Dr. Oz. "The fat buster meal to shrink your fat belly is the C.L.A. breakfast." Dr. Oz recommends eating an egg and cheese muffin with tomatoes and olive oil while taking C.L.A. capsules for breakfast for 5 days in a row. This will help get rid of the muffin top around your waist. C.L.A. (conjugated linoleic acids ) are fatty acids that naturally occur in dairy products. They are commonly used as weight loss supplements.

***Big on Top.*** "Upper body fat can be bad for your heart," warned Dr. Oz. In five days you can reduce the amount of fat in your upper body by consuming the metabolism boosting Tex Mex salad. The salad consists of spinach, corn, black beans, onion and avocado topped with salsa and sour cream. This fat buster salad is nutritious, delicious and filling. Eat the Tex Mex salad while taking an L-carnitine supplement to increase energy and reduce fat.

***Big Thighs.*** When looking for ways to reduce the fat in your thighs, Dr. Oz suggests a low-fat, high- protein diet. Have a protein shake for 5 days in place of a meal. Dr. Oz's fat buster protein shake recipe consists of bananas, blueberries, flax seeds and white kidney bean extract.

Finally, Dr. Oz presented the 'Miracle in a Bottle' to burn fat throughout the body. The miracle is raspberry ketone supplements. Raspberry ketone supplements are known to help the body burn fat. They are affordable and readily available at common health food stores.

## **Burn Fat to Lose Weight**

Many women are uncomfortable wearing a swimsuit in public because of excess weight and problem areas on their bodies. However, Dr. Oz says you can burn fat, lose weight and look great in your swimsuit with these easy additions to your diet.

***Grapefruit Juice.*** The Dr. Oz grapefruit juice drink will help your body burn fat and lose weight so you can wear your swimsuit with confidence. All you need is grapefruit juice, apple cider vinegar and honey. Simply add two teaspoons of apple cider vinegar and a spoonful of honey to a glass of grapefruit juice. Then drink this mixture every day before each meal. "It has plenty of vitamin C so it's healthy and it will burn fat," explained Dr. Oz. *(Note: If you are taking prescription medication talk to your doctor before before including grapefruit juice in your diet. Some medications cannot be taken with grapefruit juice).*

***Seaweed.*** Another beneficial food to add to your diet this summer is a type of seaweed called Nori. "It is very nutritious and will burn off fat," said Dr. Oz. Seaweed is a staple food among Asian populations known for having excellent health. Not only will seaweed support weight loss, it also has anti-aging properties.

## **The Best Frozen Foods to Lose Weight**

Dr. Oz informs dieters about the best frozen foods to lose weight. If you do not have time to prepare nutritious home cooked meals, there are plenty of healthy frozen foods available to help you lose weight. Here are 4 of Dr. Oz's favorites.

***Edamame Soybeans.*** "Frozen edamame beans are an excellent source of protein. They have about 8 grams of protein a serving," said Dr. Oz. Edamame boosts metabolism helping the body lose weight.

***Dr. Praeger's California Veggie Burgers***. Dr. Oz loves these veggie burgers because they are tasty, all-natural and contain no trans fat. They contain just over a hundred calories a serving and cost around $5.00 for a box of four frozen patties. Say goodbye to fast food burgers and hello to veggie burgers. You will lose weight and feel great.

***Trader Joe's Organic Brown Rice.*** This brown

rice is also one of the best frozen foods to lose weight. The rice is nutritious, filling and beneficial for your digestive system. "It provides about 10% of your daily fiber, which is really good," said Dr. Oz. Trader Joe's Organic Brown Rice can be prepared in 3 minutes.

***Julie's Organic Ice Cream Juliette Petite Sandwiches.*** Dr. Oz recommends these tasty treats as a way to satisfy your craving for sweets and still lose weight. These little organic ice cream sandwiches are one of the best frozen desserts to lose weight. They contain only 100 calories and 6 grams of sugar. A box of 8 costs around $5.

## Think Yourself Skinny

Do you believe it is possible to somehow use your mind to trick your body into thinking that it is full and lose weight as a result? Dr. Oz discussed the process of thinking yourself skinny with Dr. Michelle May and Dr. Gary Wenk.

According to Dr. Oz, diets usually place limits on the amount and type of food a person is permitted to eat, but the process of thinking yourself skinny does not have such restrictions. Instead, it focuses on thinking about all the foods you want to eat and eating them in your mind. Somehow this thinking process will help your body feel as if it has eaten the foods. The process used for thinking yourself skinny is known as habituation. According to Dr. Wenk, author of *Your Brain on Food*, habituation is a decreased physiological and behavioral response to repeated stimulus. Dr. May further explained that this is evidence of the mind-body connection.

Dr. Oz asked Dr. May, the author of *Eat What You Love, Love What You Eat* , to elaborate on how to think yourself skinny. Dr. May said that people are busy doing other things while they are eating, but it is important to practice mindful eating. This means eating without distractions, such as driving or talking on the telephone. Mindful eating means focusing on the task of eating, paying attention to the food, and enjoying it with all the senses. Dr. May said that when we eat without thinking, without being mindful, the brain does not properly register the food that we are eating. We also have the problem of letting ourselves get too hungry before eating. These behaviors lead us to overeat.

Dr. Oz presented a "Think Yourself Skinny" experiment that he conducted. Dr. Oz tested 2 groups of people using hidden cameras in a conference room. One group was given a bowl of candy and told to imagine eating all of it. Then they were told to eat as much of the candy as they wanted. The next group was told to imagine drinking a glass of water and then instructed to eat as much candy as they wanted. According to Dr. Oz, the group that imagined eating the candy actually ate 40% less candy than the group that imagined drinking the water. Dr. Oz's results indicated that if we visualize eating our food and awaken our senses first, we will actually eat less of the real thing. Dr. Oz reminded us that we can use the power of our minds to help us lose weight in addition to other things that we wish to accomplish.

The next time you think about starting a diet consider using your mind to control your body. Everyday before each meal imagine eating all the delicious food you love and then go for it. You will probably end up eating less, learning first hand that you have the power to think yourself skinny.

## **Lap Band Surgery**

Lap band surgery is an option that many people are choosing in an effort to lose weight. The FDA has lowered the body fat ratio and weight requirements making more people eligible for lap band surgery. This FDA change has caused controversy among medical professionals.

Dr. Oz explained the requirements for lap band surgery which was originally designed for people with extreme obesity. The FDA has now approved the surgery for people who are only 30 pounds overweight provided they have an existing health condition like high blood pressure or diabetes.

Guest doctors on the Dr. Oz show debated about the benefits and consequences of lap band surgery (gastric banding surgery). "There are a lot of complications that can arise from the lap band and they can be life threatening," warned Dr. Diana Zuckerman, who does not approve of the FDA changes, "It is difficult to take the lap band out when there are problems. Removing it is much harder than doing the surgery."

According to Dr. Louis Aronne, another guest on the Dr. Oz show, about 600,000 people around the world have the lap band and on average there has been about a 20 percent weight loss that has been maintained over a 6 year period. Dr. Aronne stated that this information was discussed at the FDA hearings. Dr. Aronne supports the FDA changes and believes that lap band surgery will help a lot of people.

There is no magic cure for obesity. Even with lap band surgery people need to take personal responsibility for their weight. More importantly, they need to understand the side-effects and possible complications of lap band surgery. Dr. Oz discussed some of the concerns with prospective lap band surgery patients and with a few people who have already had the procedure.

One side-effect of lap band surgery is acid reflux. Acid reflux could become a chronic condition that requires life-long medication. Other complications often experienced after lap band surgery are difficulty swallowing and vomiting. Two guests currently with the lap band stated that they are pleased with the results and believe that the benefits of the surgery outweigh the risks. Dr. Oz also sees the benefit of the procedure. "I think the lap band device is a remarkably effective tool," said Dr. Oz.

Undergoing weight loss surgery or any surgery is serious and could result in complications. It is best to lose weight on your own by maintaining a healthy diet and exercising daily. Consider lap band surgery as a last resort to conquer obesity.

# Part 3

# Dr. Oz

# on

# Alternative Medicine

Not all medical doctors support the use of alternative medicine. However, Dr. Oz thinks it is important to keep an open mind and urges the medical profession to be receptive to alternative treatments including herbs and supplements, acupuncture, massage, chiropractic treatment and meditation. Dr. Mimi Guarneri from Scripps Hospital, who has appeared on the Dr. Oz show, shares similar views. She is an advocate of both acupuncture and prayer – whatever works for her patients.

Dr. Oz believes there are many benefits of

acupuncture treatment and says millions of people find it to be effective. Dr. Guarneri recommends acupuncture for her patients for pain relief and to treat inflammation because it enables them to exercise and helps their hearts.

According to Dr. Oz, more than 50% of Americans use dietary supplements, such as herbs, which he and Dr. Guarneri believe are effective. Even so, it is still important to inform your doctor of any herbs and supplements you are taking and to avoid mixing them with prescription drugs and other medications.

Many patients are afraid to talk to their doctors about alternative medicine because they are not sure their doctors will be open to such practices. However, Dr. Oz recommends being personally involved in your health care and customizing therapy to meet your individual need - doing what makes sense for you.

When it comes to your health care do not be afraid to speak up or to get a second opinion. If you would like to try alternative medicine and your doctor opposes it might be time to find another doctor. After all, it is your body and your life. Modern medicine is great, but there are always risks and side-effects. Sometimes a new approach, such as acupuncture, could be perfect for your needs.

## **Acupuncture**

Dr. Oz encourages people dealing with pain to give acupuncture and other alternative therapies a try.

Chronic pain is at an all time high among people of various ages. Acupuncture could prove to be the solution. These days many people are becoming cautious of taking pain medicine on a regular basis because of the possibility of addiction and the negative side-effects.

"Acupuncture has helped my pain almost immediately," said a guest on the Dr. Oz show.

Some people fear needles and believe that acupuncture is painful, but in reality, acupuncture is not painful. Most people do not even feel the needles being inserted.

"I think acupuncture is worth trying," added Dr. Oz. "If anyone finds it uncomfortable, the acupuncturist could simply remove the needles. At least you don't have to worry about side-effects," said Dr. Oz.

Acupuncture is used to treat all types of chronic pain and is endorsed by the Cancer Centers of America as a supportive cancer therapy.

## **Acupuncture for Cancer**

Acupuncture is now recommended as a valuable treatment for cancer and continues to gain popularity in treating a variety of other chronic illnesses. Throughout Asia cancer is treated using a holistic approach which combines aspects of western medicine with acupuncture and traditional Chinese herbal medicine.

The western world has started to recognize acupuncture as an effective and beneficial treatment for cancer because it reduces the side-effects, symptoms and pain that occur with conventional cancer treatment. In fact, the Cancer Treatment Centers of America have licensed acupuncture physicians on staff at each of its five hospitals across the country.

In addition to focusing on cancer, acupuncture physicians at the Cancer Treatment Centers of America use acupuncture to treat other conditions including chronic fatigue, hot flashes, anxiety, stress and pain. Some acupuncturists at the cancer centers focus specifically on reducing the side-effects of standard cancer treatment - radiation, chemotherapy and surgery.

Acupuncture is beneficial to the overall well-being of people suffering with cancer. Research indicates that acupuncture is effective in supporting the immune system, which could help the body fight cancer. Moreover, acupuncture enhances the mood of cancer patients, increases their energy levels and helps them sleep better. In other words, acupuncture improves the quality of life for people battling cancer.

More cancer specialists are starting to recommend acupuncture for their cancer patients. They believe that using acupuncture simultaneously with chemotherapy, radiation and surgery is the best form of treatment for cancer patients because it eliminates pain without the use of drugs and reduces the degree of other side-effects.

People currently undergoing treatment for cancer should talk to their doctors about using acupuncture as a complementary cancer treatment. It is easy to locate a licensed acupuncture physician by contacting the National Certification Commission for Acupuncture and Oriental Medicine (NCCAOM).

## **Alternative Treatments for Pain**

Alternative treatments for pain play an important role in the field of medicine. "Alternative treatments are extremely cost effective and could be done in the comfort of your home. My wife uses homeopathic therapies with our kids," stated Dr. Oz. "I am not an alternative medicine doctor, but I do know something about it. I use arnica for pain, bruises and sprains."

Homeopathic therapies focus on helping the body heal itself. Although some modern medical doctors question natural treatments, there are studies that indicate effectiveness. Homeopathic alternative treatments involve using small doses of medicine to send messages to the body, so that the body is then triggered to begin healing itself.

Dr. Oz stated that homeopathic treatments could be safer than conventional medicine because it uses such a small amount of medication. "Conventional medications can affect your kidneys and other organs. Homeopathic therapies don't do that," explained Dr. Oz.

For common pain such as a stiff neck Dr. Oz recommends using heat instead of cold packs because cold packs tend to make the muscles stiff. There is no need to buy heating pads. You can make an effective heating pad at home. "Take a sock and fill it with uncooked rice and add a few drops of lavender oil . Tie the sock on the end and then heat it in the microwave," said Dr. Oz.

Dr. Lee Wolfer, a graduate of Harvard Medical School appeared on the Dr. Oz show. Dr. Wolfer uses a relatively new alternative cure, biopuncture, to treat patients suffering from intense pain. "I've been able to achieve results with biopuncture that I was never able to achieve before," she told Dr. Oz. "I get great results with my patients. Most have tried a lot of options and medicines for pain that did not work."

## **Medical Marijuana**

The use of medical marijuana was the topic of a heated debate on an episode of the Dr. Oz show. "Fifteen states and Washington D.C. have legalized the use of medical marijuana," said Dr. Oz. He further stated that the use of marijuana for medical purposes goes back well over 200 years until the government made it an illegal, controlled substance.

"How many of you think medical marijuana should be legalized," Dr. Oz asked his audience. Approximately 75% of the audience members raised their hands. "That is about the same as the national average," replied Dr. Oz.

Dr. Oz then welcomed talk show host, author and entrepreneur, Montel Williams to speak about the issue of medical marijuana. Montel was diagnosed with multiple sclerosis and remains a strong advocate for using marijuana for medical reasons. "The pain was so bad that I used to take up to 8 Oxycontin pills a day. The drugs started to affect my health, my kidneys. Medical marijuana was the only thing that has helped me. It has given me my life back," insisted Montel Williams.

"I have seen the pain you've endured. Multiple sclerosis is when your immune system goes crazy and it causes intense pain," said Dr. Oz.

Not only has medical marijuana given Montel Williams a much needed break from the pain of his illness, it has also helped the disease itself. "I have not had one additional plaque form on my MRIs since I started using medical marijuana," said Williams.

"Two leading medical groups have stated that medical marijuana should be legal," said Dr. Oz. He then welcomed two medical doctors to speak about medical marijuana - Dr. Andrea Barthwell, who is against using marijuana for medical purposes, and Dr. Donald Abrams, who supports its use. Dr. Barthwell stated that she cannot support the smoking of marijuana and believes that if it is legalized the use of it would go up, especially among younger people.

Dr. Oz asked Dr. Abrams why he supports the use of medical marijuana. "I am a cancer specialist," replied Dr. Donald Abrams, "I deal with people who are in extreme pain and dying. I support the use of medical marijuana because it helps them. It is an inhaled drug, just like other medications." Dr. Abrams and Montel Williams further explained that doctors and patients should make the decisions about their medical treatment. "We want to get the government out of the doctor-patient relationship," said Williams.

"I think medical marijuana makes sense when using

it to treat certain conditions like chronic pain, glaucoma and cancer," said Dr. Oz. "I've gone to medical school to learn how to be a doctor, to treat patients, and sometimes the system pisses me off. Who should get between me treating my patient who cannot get relief any other way?" he asked. "No one," replied some guests and audience members who support the use of medical marijuana.

"I used to have severe seizures. It was so bad that I really had no life. They even took my driver's license. Medication was not helping me. Finally, one doctor suggested that marijuana might help me," said a female audience member. "I have not had one seizure in 8 years since I started medical marijuana. I no longer have to use it and I've never had any symptoms of withdrawal. I'm with Montel on this. It has given me back my life. I am a productive member of society, " she insisted.

Dr. Andrea Barthwell along with a few others voiced opposing views and concerns about addiction. Dr. Oz countered with, "How come cigarettes are legal when we know that tobacco is addictive and so are many other medicines?" This was the million dollar question that no one seemed to be able to answer.

"Medical marijuana should be used to give patients their life back, not to take away their lives," said Dr. Oz.

## **The Hero of Alternative Medicine**

Dr. Joseph Mercola, also known as the hero of alternative medicine, shared his views about medicine. Dr. Oz's burning question was "Why are you so controversial?" Dr. Mercola explained that he is passionate about getting people healthy while many other doctors are just interesting in treating diseases.

"I focus on natural ways to get people healthy, and everyone else is focusing on a magic pill," stated Dr. Joseph Mercola. "We only sell natural products. No one could ever die from the natural supplements we sell - the natural food based substances." Dr. Mercola further explained that "over 100,000 people die each year from properly prescribed drugs," while emphasizing the importance of using natural approaches.

Dr. Mercola has been criticized for his medical practices and beliefs about medicine. Many western doctors oppose his views. According to Dr. Mercola, there is a lot of information about health and medicine that doctors do not want the public to know about. He asserts that many people are sick because of their doctors. "People want health and relief. In many cases the traditional model has failed them."

Dr. Mercola shared a few alternative medical breakthroughs. "Coconut oil may be useful in the treatment and prevention of Alzheimer's, which is good because we have an Alzheimer's epidemic," said Dr. Mercola. Dr. Oz followed by saying that this "does not sound as dangerous as other treatment methods." Dr. Mercola further discussed the health benefits of L-Arginine, an amino acid that helps with blood flow improvement, and Astaxanthin, a cousin to beta-carotene that he states is "the most potent antioxidant that we know of. Odds are you can likely prevent cataracts with Astaxanthin."

Dr. Oz is open-minded when it comes to alternative medicine and he embraces many elements of alternative and natural health methods. Unfortunately, Dr. Oz has been criticized by many doctors of drug-based medicine for providing a forum for holistic doctors who support natural health.

Dr. Joseph Mercola is a licensed osteopathic physician and surgeon who received his medical training at the Chicago College of Osteopathic Medicine and completed residency at Chicago Osteopathic Hospital. He is qualified and trained to prescribe drugs and perform surgery. He is also board certified in family medicine. Dr. Mercola is dedicated to healing the body instead of simply treating isolated symptoms. He prefers to use natural approaches to health because he believes they are healthier and much safer for the body.

Alternative medicine has a long, solid history which spans thousands of years in the eastern world. Treatments such as acupuncture, yoga, natural food products, herbs and plant-based diets have proved effective. However, most drug-focused doctors in the United States, are quick to criticize practices that they do not understand, cannot prove based on the scientific method, and medical practices or medicine that they cannot patent.

# Part 4

# Dr. Oz on Anti-Aging

### Anti-Aging Tips

Follow the anti-aging tips of Dr. Oz to improve your overall health and well-being. Basic products and simple lifestyle changes could add years to your life while making you look and feel younger.

***Eliminate Exhaustion.*** Dr. Oz recommends getting proper rest and an adequate amount of sleep each night as a priority for anti-aging success. Lack of sleep causes the body to age. Most people do not get the amount of rest needed to heal and revitalize the body.

***Add Spice.*** According to Dr. Oz, spices such as ginger, cayenne pepper, and cinnamon can do wonders for your health. Many people experience arthritis in the aging process. Ginger spice is known to alleviate arthritic pain. Both ginger and cayenne pepper are useful for lowering high blood pressure and cinnamon helps lower cholesterol and blood sugar levels.

***Take Vitamins.*** Americans have one of the worst diets on the planet, which contains too much fat, sugar and salt while lacking in nutrients. Insufficient nutrition will cause your body to age. Dr. Oz's anti-aging remedy is to take a daily multivitamin, especially if you have poor eating habits. Also take steps to improve your diet by increasing your intake of vegetables, fruits and whole grains.

***Exercise.*** Another important anti-aging remedy is regular exercise. Exercise is necessary to strengthen the body and to help eliminate stress. Dr. Oz recommends exercising a minimum of three times each week.

***Minimize Wrinkles.*** Moisturizing your skin will help reduce the appearance of wrinkles. Dr. Oz offers a home-remedy known as the Botox substitute. Simply mix a small mashed banana with 2 ounces of plain yogurt and a spoonful of honey. Apply the mixture to your face and leave on for 15 to 20 minutes. Then gently rinse the mask from your face. Your skin will look and feel wonderful. This is a great and effective treatment. It is cheap, easy to do and has no known side-effects.

## **Botox Considerations**

Botox can be dangerous. Dr. Oz discussed the controversy of one of the most common cosmetic procedures requested by women to reduce the appearance of wrinkles and increase fullness in the lips.

***If your Botox is too cheap, it could be fake.*** Due to an increased demand in Botox injections, the supply of cheap, fake, mail-order Botox is on the rise. Be careful ordering do-it-yourself Botox injection kits through the Internet. You could end up with a fake product that results in serious injury or death.

***Store front Botox clinics could be dangerous.*** It is best to use a reputable and licensed health care facility for all your cosmetic procedures. It is not uncommon to find illegal Botox clinics advertising special discounts. Do not fall prey to a scam that not only takes your money, but also places your health in danger.

***Ask the right questions.*** According to Dr. Oz it is essential to have the right answers to the following questions when considering Botox:

*1-Who will be injecting it?*

*2-What kind of Botox is it?*

*3-Where will you go to get the injections?*

Make sure that a licensed plastic surgeon or dermatologist will give the injections. Ask to see the bottle to make sure it is sealed and labeled Allergan Cosmetics and check the expiration date. Only agree to get Botox injections in a doctor's office. You may also wish to consider researching to find out how long the practice has been there and to learn more about the doctor. When it comes to your health you can never be too careful.

## Look Younger

"Skin is the main thing that shows your age" warned Dr. Oz. Therefore, if you want to defy your age and look younger you have to take good care of your skin. The first step to younger looking skin is to get rid of brown spots and to minimize crows feet. This alone will take years off the appearance of your skin.

Another simple step you can take to defy age is to drink a daily "fountain of youth shake," said Dr. Oz. Prepare the shake by mixing coconut water with spinach, pineapple, green apples and ginger. Then add a few wheatgrass ice cubes and blend. This drink is rich in antioxidants and will prevent wrinkles from forming so your skin will look younger.

Finally, you can look younger based on the clothing you wear. "Put your clothes on a diet," stated Dr. Oz. It is important for women to wear clothes that suit their body types. Baggy, dark colored clothing can make you look older. Wear clothes that fit and those that have color to add life.

## **HGH - Human Growth Hormone**

The human growth hormone is not the fountain of youth that people have been led to believe, according to Dr. Oz. Although HGH injections are used to enhance beauty and provide energy nothing can restore youth. Beauty and a younger-looking appearance are only skin deep. Dr. Oz warned about the dangers that occur under the surface for people using human growth hormones. "HGH will disrupt the normal hormone systems of the body leading to all kinds of health problems. It could even cause cancer." In addition to the cancer risk HGH may increase the risk of heart disease and diabetes.

Despite the known health dangers of HGH, some medical doctors and other health professionals continue to promote and support the use of HGH. Some people are even getting human growth hormone injections from people outside the medical field and ordering HGH from the Internet. "People need to be careful. HGH is serious and the consequences of using it are serious. People using HGH are one big experiment like mice in cages. We do not know the long-term outcome of this hormone," explained Dr. Oz.

In addition, Dr. Oz said that the medical profession does not always make decisions that are best for patients or the public and urges people to be aware of this fact. "With HGH the trade-off is not worth it," he insisted.

# Part 5

# Dr. Oz

# on

# Healthy Living

### Boost Your Immune System

Boost your immune system by eating the right foods. Dr. Oz recommends 5 foods that will strengthen your immunity to help your body resist and fight illnesses.

***Garlic***. Garlic is a top food choice of Dr. Oz for boosting the immune system. Garlic contains powerful antioxidants and other substances that ward off diseases. Including fresh garlic in your recipes will not only increase your immunity, but it will enhance the flavor of your food.

***Miso Soup***. Miso soup has "antibacterial properties and boosts antibodies in the bloodstream," advises Dr. Oz. Miso is actually a type of fermented soybean paste. Miso soup also contains seaweed and tofu. It is a favorite among Asian cultures.

***Papaya-Carrot Juice***. This is the perfect juice combination for boosting the immune system, according to Dr. Oz. Papaya-carrot juice is rich in beta-carotene (vitamin A), which builds white blood cells and helps the body fight infections. Sweet potatoes are another excellent source of vitamin A.

***Elderberry Juice.*** "Elderberry juice has antiviral properties that help block the flu virus," explained Dr. Oz. Elderberry juice is known to boost immunity and relieve cold and flu symptoms. Elderberry juice can be purchased at health food stores. It also comes as a supplement in the form of capsules.

***Sardines***. Dr. Oz recommends eating sardines to boost the immune system. Sardines are rich in vitamin D, which protects against infections. If you do not like the taste of sardines, simply spend 15 minutes a day in the sun so your body can produce its own vitamin D.

## **Supercharge Your Health**

Supercharge your health with the help of Dr. Oz. Eat better, sleep better and feel better by following the advice of America's favorite doctor.

***Supercharge Your Metabolism.*** If you are having difficulty losing weight, your metabolism could be sluggish. Taking a cold shower for 5 minutes is a great way to supercharge your metabolism and improve your feeling of health and wellness.

***Supercharge Your Mood.*** Good bacteria in the body helps produce serotonin which improves mood. A tasty and nutritious way to get good bacteria is to eat kimchi, a traditional Korean food made from cabbage and spicy red pepper. Dr. Oz encourages health conscious consumers to try new foods. We can learn a lot from Asian populations known for their excellent health and longevity.

***Supercharge Your Sleep.*** Are you tossing and turning during the night? Do you fail to get enough sleep? Dr. Oz shares a simple secret to better sleep - butter before bedtime. Eating 2 spoons of almond butter before bedtime will stabilize blood sugar levels improving the quality of sleep, thus supporting good health.

## **Take Vitamins**

In addition to eating a healthy diet, Dr. Oz recommends taking a combination of daily vitamins and nutritional supplements to maintain overall health and wellness. Three top choices of Dr. Oz are multivitamins, a vitamin C supplement and a vitamin D supplement.

***Multivitamins***. According to Dr. Oz, a multi-vitamin should be taken everyday. He recommends breaking the vitamin in two and taking half in the morning and the other half in the evening. Dr. Oz says this will help the body to absorb the vitamins better while reducing the likelihood of getting an upset stomach which sometimes occurs when taking vitamins. Multivitamins increase energy, help with memory problems and strengthen the immune system.

***Vitamin C***. Known for its ability to boost immunity, vitamin C is a favorite of Dr. Oz. Vitamin C is a powerful antioxidant that supports the health of the eyes, bones and skin. It reduces the risks for heart disease and urinary tract infections. More importantly, vitamin C helps the body absorb other important nutrients. Dr. Oz recommends taking a supplement or drinking a glass of fresh orange juice each day.

**Vitamin D**. Another favorite supplement of Dr. Oz is vitamin D which is also known for its ability to boost immunity. As a matter of fact, Dr. Oz believes that vitamin D could actually be more important than vitamin C in strengthening the immune system. Vitamin D is known for supporting bone health and helping reduce inflammation in the body. Additionally, vitamin D may help prevent many types of cancer.

## 7 Day Energy Surge

If you are suffering from constant fatigue and could use a double dose of energy perhaps you should try the 7 day energy surge. Weight loss expert and author of the book *"The 7 Day Energy Surge,"* Jim Karas and Dr. Oz presented a 4-step plan to restore energy in the body.

**Makeover the Morning.** How you start your mornings will affect your energy level for the rest of the day.

Based on *The 7 Day Energy Surge*, it is recommended that you remain in bed for 10 minutes after waking each morning. During this time do simple breathing exercises to increase the oxygen levels in your body. Then get out of bed, open the curtains and turn on the light. The light will reprogram your circadian rhythm to alert your body that sleep time has ended. Next, eat a healthy breakfast that is rich in protein and fiber.

**Take a Vitamin Cocktail**. The second step on t*The Sevy Energy Surge* is the vitamin cocktail, which is composed of magnesium and tyrosine supplements. Taking these supplements will help increase energy levels in the body which is often depleted by stress, insufficient rest, poor eating habits and other factors. The recommendation is 400 mg of magnesium and 500 mg of tyrosine.

**Upgrade the Afternoon Snack.** Dr Oz and Jim Karas point out the importance of having a healthy afternoon energy booster instead of the usual soda, coffee or candy. They recommend wheat grass for the energy surge you need. Not only does wheat grass increase energy, but it also protects the body from illnesses due to its high levels of antioxidants. Wheat grass can usually be purchased at health food stores and juice bars. It is also available as a supplement.

***Prepare for Sleep.*** The final step of the *7 Day Energy Surge* is making your bedroom environment conducive to sleep. This means going to bed at the same time each night and eliminating detractors of sleep, such as television and phones. Prior to bedtime you should lower the lights, relax and wind down. Chronic health conditions are linked to poor sleep quality. Thus, sleeping well is essential for optimum health and energy.

## How to Stop Smoking

Learn how to stop smoking by learning to love yourself, advises Dr. Oz, who believes that it is virtually impossible to quit smoking cigarettes without developing strong self-love.

"I never tell anyone to stop smoking. There is a zero percent chance that it will work," said Dr. Oz. "I say love yourself. When you love yourself you will not want to smoke," insisted Dr. Oz.

Dr. Oz shared the philosophy that people who really

love themselves will not continue to do things to harm themselves. They will find ways to overcome.

Currently, more than 20% of adults in the United States smoke cigarettes. Smoking is an expensive addiction that leads to a myriad of serious health problems, including lung cancer. Making the decision to quit smoking can save your life. The question is, *"Do you love yourself enough to quit?"*

## **The Dr. Oz Weekend Challenge**

Take the weekend challenge so you can get off to a great start Monday morning. Dr. Oz explained the perfect 2-day health plan to rejuvenate and energize your body and mind. Dr. Oz believes his weekend challenge is the solution to conquer the dreaded Monday morning blues that we experience before heading back to work each week. The plan is painless and easy to implement.

***Get Up Early.*** Dr. Oz challenges us to get up early on the weekend instead of sleeping late. Most people sleep late on weekends which usually makes it more difficult to get up early come Monday. Force yourself to get up early on the weekends until it becomes a habit.

***Limit Alcoholic Beverages.*** Many people social with family and friends on the weekends. As you relax and unwind, remember to limit your intake of alcoholic beverages. Dr. Oz said to "rethink your drink and detox your appetizers." Limit yourself to 2 glasses of wine and opt for healthier appetizers, such as fresh vegetables.

***Shop Sunday Night.*** Dr. Oz's weekend challenge calls for shopping on Sunday nights. The best deals are Sunday nights. The store will be less crowded, which means it will be less stressful to shop and you'll save money on the deals. Remember to check the higher and lower shelves for items priced at a discount. Stock up on produce and healthy foods so you can pack a nutritious lunch during the week.

***Home Health Renovation.*** Another step on the Dr. Oz weekend challenge is the home health renovation. Dr. Oz recommends finding natural ways to deal with minor health issues. Leave the pain medicine in the cabinet and give yourself acupressure for headaches, which are usually the result of stress. For constipation, forget about laxatives. Dr. Oz urges us to eat more fiber. Most people get about half the amount of the fiber they need each day. Be careful taking antibiotics. "If you are taking antibiotics that you don't need you are risking your life," said Dr. Oz

***Healthy Sunday Dinner.*** "Monday morning is the most common time when people have heart attacks," said Dr. Oz. He suggests eating a heart healthy dinner on Sunday evening - vegetables, whole grains and fresh fruit, such as kiwi and strawberries, which helps lower cholesterol levels.

## Live to Be 100

Dr. Oz explains how we can live to be 100 years old by sharing the secrets of the fountain of youth, things that help us live longer. Most people that live to be 100 maintain a lifestyle somewhat different from the rest of us. They make healthier lifestyle choices.

***Attitude***. Believe it or not your attitude will affect just how long you could live, so be optimistic. People who have a positive attitude live longer. They have less stress and a stronger immune system. They also have more energy because negativity saps your energy. Your attitude not only influences the length of your life, but it plays a role in how successful you become. More importantly, your attitude will determine the quality of your relationships with other people.

***Exercise***. Exercise is essential to a long and healthy life. If you want to live to be 100 years old then you need to make exercise a daily habit. Exercise will strengthen your muscles and joints, relieve stress and give you energy. Exercise will lower your blood pressure which reduces your risk of heart attack and stroke.

***Interests***. Having interests that stimulate your brain is essential for people striving to live to the age of 100. Your brain needs challenging tasks. Crossword puzzles help. Learning a new language or taking an advanced math class will probably do more. Find something in which you are interested that provides a challenging learning process.

***Nutrition***. Diet is important to overall health and longevity. If your are suffering from obesity, chances are you will not live to be 100 years old. Eat a healthy diet rich in vegetables, fruits, and whole grains. Lose the excess weight.

***Quit Smoking***. It is almost impossible to find a smoker who has lived to be 100 years old. Smoking could reduce your life expectancy by as much as 15 years. Smoking weakens your immune system and leads to all kinds of respiratory illnesses. It might be easier to quit if you remember that every time you light a cigarette you are burning days off of your life.

# Part 6

# Dr. Oz

# on

# Medical Conditions

**<u>Chronic Fatigue Syndrome</u>**

Thanks to Dr. Oz chronic fatigue syndrome is now seen as a real disease and not just a figment of the imagination. Thousands of people, mostly women, suffer with chronic fatigue syndrome. It interferes with their livelihood, peace of mind and quality of life. Dr. Oz has helped bring attention and awareness to chronic fatigue syndrome, which has often been dismissed by other medical doctors. People suffering with the disease have often been left to face the challenges on their own.

***What is chronic fatigue syndrome?*** Chronic fatigue syndrome is a serious condition which causes a person to remain in a state of exhaustion. The exhaustion is further exacerbated by mental and physical activity. To make matters worse, chronic fatigue syndrome usually does not improve with bed rest. Most people with chronic fatigue syndrome wake up already feeling exhausted. They usually suffer with poor concentration, muscle aches and headaches. Dr. Oz stated that people with chronic fatigue syndrome feel as if they have the flu that never goes away.

***What causes chronic fatigue syndrome?*** Doctors are not sure of the exact cause of this condition. According to Dr. Oz, anemia and hypothyroidism are both contributors to chronic fatigue syndrome. If you have anemia it is important to increase your iron intake. This is best accomplished by eating iron rich foods such as broccoli and spinach. It is also beneficial to use iron cookware. Talk with your doctor before taking iron supplements which lead to constipation or other problems if taken in excess. If hypothyroidism is responsible for your chronic fatigue symptoms, discuss treatment options with your doctor. In the meantime, eat a healthy, well-balanced diet rich in vitamins and nutrients to increase your energy level. Also consider taking magnesium supplements. "Magnesium will help your body convert food into energy," said Dr. Oz.

Chronic fatigue syndrome often leads to other health problems such as depression, high blood pressure and weight gain. Do not suffer in silence. If you are constantly exhausted seek treatment.

## **Hysterectomy and Fibroids**

"A hysterectomy is usually unnecessary as a treatment for fibroids " warned Dr. Oz. Unfortunately, many women undergo this risky surgery when less invasive options are available. Fibroids are usually benign, although they could result in discomfort or heavy menstrual periods.

***Hysterectomy Risks***. Dr. Oz advises women to research all available options before making the decision to have a hysterectomy for fibroids. "It is the number one surgery that women have that they usually don't need." Having a hysterectomy could also be life-threatening.

Hundreds of women who entered the hospital for hysterectomies did not come out alive and some of those who did survive the surgery and hospital stay later died from resulting complications.

Hysterectomy is casually recommended by many doctors as a normal treatment for fibroids, However, it should actually be the last resort. Dr. Oz supports hysterectomy in cases of already life-threatening conditions, such as uterine cancer.

***Fibroid Symptoms***. Up to 80% of women will have fibroids by the age of forty. In many cases the fibroids will not have symptoms. However, fibroids could cause back pain or put pressure on the bladder causing frequent urges to urinate. In rare cases fibroids could interfere with fertility. As women transition through menopause, fibroids usually stop growing and start to shrink. In most cases, medical intervention, especially hysterectomy, is not necessary for fibroids.

***Treatment Options***. Other treatment options for fibroids presented by Dr. Oz include myomectomy and anti-estrogen therapy. Myomectomy is surgical procedure that removes each individual fibroid while leaving the woman's complete reproductive system intact. Anti-estrogen therapy involves using hormone blockers to keep the ovaries from producing estrogen causing the fibroids to shrink.

***Acupuncture.*** For women seeking a natural treatment for fibroids, acupuncture may be the best option. Research has demonstrated that acupuncture has been effective in stopping the growth of fibroids and shrinking existing fibroid tumors. Dr. Oz supports acupuncture as a beneficial natural therapy for a variety of health issues.

## **Preventing Alzheimer's**

Breakthrough medical research linking Alzheimer's disease directly to the foods we eat was presented on the Dr. Oz show. It turns out that our diets may influence our risks for Alzheimer's more than genetic factors. This offers new hope for people with a family history of Alzheimer's who fear they might eventually develop the disease.

"I think we can prevent Alzheimer's just by what we eat," said Dr. Oz. There is no doubt that diet influences our overall health, but that influence is greater than many people realize. A healthy diet is essential in preventing many diseases. "Alzheimer's is not just caused from your genes. The foods you eat might trigger Alzheimer's." warned Dr. Oz.

Dr. Suzanne Delamonte, a leading medical researcher, described Alzheimer's as diabetes of the brain. Dr. Oz agreed that "having diabetes or prediabetes increases your chances of developing Alzheimer's." Dr. Delamonte further explained that diabetes can take place anywhere in the body. It can occur in the muscles, the liver and in the brain.

Dr. Richard Carmona, an expert on brain research, also spoke about diet being a major factor in the development of Alzheimer's. "People that are overweight have higher incidence of Alzheimer's," stated Dr. Carmona, who explained that the quality of our food is significant. "Stay away from nitrates. Start eating organic. Eat foods with the least amount of preservatives." Dr. Carmona admitted to Dr. Oz that he would not eat any foods that contain sodium nitrates or nitrites. Dr. Suzanne Delamonte confirmed that sodium nitrates contribute to brain insulin resistance.

"Chemicals from the foods we eat everyday cause problems. Smoked meats are a big problem," warned Dr. Oz. Although many processed foods contain sodium nitrates and nitrites, the ingredients are listed on the labels so you will know which foods to avoid. However, beer could be a problem. "The ingredients for beer are not listed on beer labels so you need to be careful with beer," said Dr. Oz.

Take responsibility for your health. You have the power to control what goes into your body. Read the labels. Avoid eating foods that contain harmful chemicals and preservatives.

**Sciatica**

Age related changes to the spine are one of the most common causes of sciatica, according to Dr. Oz. Sciatica pain is an indication that the nerves in the spinal column are pinched due to compressed disks in the spine. Sciatica pain, which is often severe, can strike without warning. It usually occurs in the lower back and legs, but it could cause pain throughout the entire body.

Dr. Oz shares 2 natural treatments that could help relieve sciatica pain. The first is a stretching exercise. Lie flat on your back while raising your knees towards your head. Try to touch your chin with your knees in order to stretch out the lower back. Initially, there will be pain in doing this exercise, but over time it will help with sciatica.

The second natural treatment to help with sciatic nerve pain is to use heat. Dr. Oz recommends using a heated back massager. Heat relaxes and soothes muscles and joints helping to reduce pain and discomfort. Place a heated massager in your favorite chair and use it regularly to treat sciatica.

If you are unable to deal with sciatica pain on your own, but are not interested in taking medication or having surgery, seek natural treatment from a holistic health care professional. Natural treatment, such as acupuncture, is highly recommended.

***Acupuncture for Sciatica.*** Treating sciatic nerve pain with acupuncture involves inserting hair-thin needles into the skin at specific points on the body. The procedure is not painful and does not have the side-effects associated with conventional treatment.

## Women's Depression

Depression in women is misdiagnosed up to 50% of the time, according to Dr. Oz. While nearly 17 million

Americans suffer depression each year, women are twice as likely as men to become depressed. Dr. Oz says that hormones, menstrual cycles, pregnancy and menopause are all factors which make women more likely to experience depression.

Severe depression often calls for medical intervention. Depression makes it difficult to maintain a normal life. It affects all aspects of a person's life, including the ability to eat, sleep and concentrate. According to Dr. Oz, treatment for depression is effective in relieving symptoms most of the time.

Sometimes it is difficult to tell whether depression is the problem or if a person is simply facing some challenges which cause a bad mood. Thus, it is important to know the warning signs of depression and to seek assistance if needed. Dr. Oz identifies several signs of depression. Symptoms of depression include loss of interest in normal activities, changes in appetite, changes in sleeping habits and constant feelings of sadness. Additionally, if the people around you think that you are depressed, you probably are.

Dr. Oz advises taking the following steps to help

overcome depression. After seeking medical assistance, work on getting enough sleep, exercising daily and eating properly. Get plenty of sunlight and consume foods rich in omega-3 fatty acids. Finally, surround yourself with a positive support system.

## **Heart Attack**

Heart attacks are the leading cause of death in America, but they could be prevented. Dr. Oz gave pertinent advice on "how to prevent a heart attack in 28 days." Dr. Oz's action plan for preventing heart attack includes doing artery maintenance for your heart, strengthening your heart, lowering your blood pressure and reducing stress.

***Artery Maintenance.*** According to Dr. Oz, keeping your arteries clean is an important step in heart attack prevention. This means preventing plaque buildup and blood clots. Dr. Oz stated that poor eating habits and lack of exercise contribute to clogged arteries which leads to heart attacks. Therefore, it is important to exercise daily and make healthy food choices. Dr. Oz recommends starting with basic exercise, such as simple stretching. He also recommends including flax seed oil in your diet and taking 2 baby aspirin tablets every evening to help ward off heart attacks.

***Strengthening the Heart***. Dr. Oz said the plan in this step is to increase your heart rate. Increasing your heart rate could reduce your risk of having a heart attack by 30%. Taking daily power walks and walking up and down the stairs is a great way to increase your heart rate. Likewise, work on reducing your cholesterol levels by cutting back on foods high in cholesterol, such as eggs.

***Lowering Blood Pressure***. High blood pressure, which is directly linked to heart attacks, is easy to prevent with simple lifestyle changes. Lower your blood pressure by eating plenty of vegetables, reducing your consumption of fatty meats, exercising daily, getting proper rest and remaining calm (heated arguments raise blood pressure).

***Reducing Stress***. Reducing stress helps prevent heart attacks. Stress causes physical damage to the arteries and often leads to depression. Find ways to reduce the amount of stress in your life. Exercise, yoga, meditation and even bubble baths help relieve stress. Some people find that keeping a stress journal is helpful because it makes them more aware of when stress happens giving them more control.

Do not be a victim of a heart attack. Follow the advice of Dr. Oz by spending the next 28 days making the lifestyle changes needed to prevent a heart attack.

## **Heart Attack Warning Signs**

Dr. Oz provides 5 warning signs of a heart attack that everyone should be familiar with. Heart attack is a leading cause of death in the United States. Knowing the common signs and symptoms could save your life.

***Neck Pain***. Although neck pain occurs often in people with desk jobs, Dr. Oz warns that it is a known warning sign of a heart attack. If you suddenly experience neck pain seemingly without cause seek medical assistance to rule out the onset of a heart attack.

***Unusual Fatigue***. Americans are working multiple jobs to make ends meet, so it is normal to become exhausted. However, if you are constantly feeling fatigue and you are not overworking, your fatigue is cause for concern. Dr. Oz's advice is to get a checkup. Suffering a heart attack is a real possibility.

***Nausea and Indigestion***. According to Dr. Oz, nausea and indigestion are a sign that something is amiss in your body. Prior to suffering a heart attack, people often experience both nausea and indigestion. Again, these warning signs are cause for concern.

***Shortness of Breath***. Unless you have just run a marathon or participated in other strenuous exercises, you should not be short of breath. If you are having difficulty breathing seek immediate medical assistance. Dr. Oz states that shortness of breath is one heart attack warning sign that should not be ignored.

***Dizziness and Lightheadedness***. Dizziness and lightheadedness occur when blood pressure drops too low. Sitting and elevating the feet sometimes helps. However, if you feel dizzy or lightheaded even while sitting Dr. Oz recommends seeing a doctor because these common warning signs of a heart attack are often overlooked.

## Heartburn

The pain symptoms experienced by heartburn are similar to those of someone having a heart attack, warns Dr. Oz. Therefore it is important to understand and know the difference because your life could depend on it.

According to Dr. Oz, heartburn is characterized by a painful, burning sensation just below the chest area that may move to the throat. The pain usually occurs after eating and often subsides when you move around or press against the area. Other heartburn symptoms include burping, difficulty swallowing and hoarseness. The onset of a heart attack is described as a crushing pressure in the chest that may move towards the back, neck or arms. Shortness of breath, dizziness and sweating may accompany the pain of a heart attack. If you are not sure whether you are experiencing severe heartburn or starting to have a heart attack seek immediate medical assistance.

Although millions of Americans suffer with severe heartburn, it is sometimes misdiagnosed. If you have been experiencing and treating the symptoms of heartburn for more than six months and you have frequent flare-ups, visit your doctor to rule out a more serious condition such as acid reflux disease or esophageal cancer.

***How to Treat Heartburn at Home.*** Dr. Oz recommends the use of chewable antacids to relieve the symptoms of heartburn in people who have occasional flare-ups. Chewable antacids work quickly, are inexpensive and available over-the-counter. Making dietary changes and eating smaller portions of food will also help eliminate heartburn. Ginger tea may help prevent heartburn, whereas tomato based foods, spicy foods, chocolates and coffee may trigger heartburn.

***Medical Treatment for Heartburn.*** Medical treatment is available for people suffering with severe heartburn. Treatment may include prescription drugs or surgery. However, there is the potential for increased side-effects and complications with medical intervention. If you are considering conventional medical treatment for heartburn discuss the risks and benefits with your doctor.

# Part 7

# Dr. Oz

# on

# Food and Drinks

**Organic Food is Better**

Dr. Oz insists that organic food is better for your health despite news reports to the contrary. According to Dr. Oz, the argument is not about the amount of nutrition in organic food versus conventional, non-organic food. All versions of fruits and vegetables contain comparable amounts of vitamins and nutrients. The issue, says Dr. Oz, is that non-organic food is high in toxic chemicals, like pesticides, that are dangerous to health. In addition to the high levels of pesticides in non-organic food, these foods also contain antibiotics, synthetic hormones, genetically modified organisms (GMOs) and irradiation. Organic food is free of this making it better for your body.

"There are 4 types of foods that you should definitely eat organic, even if that means paying higher prices," asserts Dr. Oz

**Potatoes**. "With potatoes you get a double dose of harmful stuff," said Dr. Oz. "First, the potato vines are sprayed with chemical pesticides and then the potatoes absorb harmful things, including fungus from the soil." Dr. Oz further explained that sweet potatoes contain less pesticides than white potatoes. "If you can not afford organic potatoes then it's best to eat sweet potatoes."

**Celery and Peppers**. If you regularly include celery and peppers in your diet you should switch to organic brands. These two vegetables are high in pesticide and it is difficult to wash off.

**Leafy Greens**. "Spinach, lettuce and collard greens are best in organic varieties. They could cost up to 50% more, but they really are better for your health."

***Dairy Products***. Dr. Oz warns that dairy products, which are consumed daily in the average American diet, should always be eaten organic. "This includes milk, ice cream, butter, yogurt, and cheese." Conventional dairy products contain harmful ingredients, including antibiotics and hormones, that negatively affect health.

## Herbal Tea

Healing herbal teas provide instant relief from everyday ailments. Dr. Oz explained the benefits of healing herbal teas, which are effective in treating a variety of common health conditions. Herbal teas do not cause the harmful side-effects found in most traditional medicine. Before opening the medicine cabinet reach for your tea kettle so you can enjoy a natural herbal tea treatment.

***Sage Tea.*** According to Dr. Oz, "Sage herbal tea is the best tea for improving your mood." Sage has a long history of being used to treat a multitude of health problems. Some studies have indicated that sage herbal tea helps improve memory in people with Alzheimer's disease and it could help stabilize blood sugar levels in some diabetic patients. Other healing properties of sage herbal tea include relieving anxiety, soothing sore throats, alleviating menstruation problems, reducing menopause symptoms and healing cuts.

**Rooibos Tea.** Another herbal tea that provides instant relief is rooibos tea. According to Dr. Oz, "Rooibos is the best tea for irritated skin." Rooibos is high in nutrients and vitamins, and is beneficial for overall health. This herbal tea helps heal skin conditions such as acne and eczema. Drinking rooibos tea or applying it topically to the skin helps minimize skin breakouts. Rooibos tea contains anti-aging properties. It neutralizes free-radicals in the skin, which slows down the aging process. Using rooibos tea is definitely a first step to healthier, younger-looking skin.

**Nettle Tea.** If you are suffering from allergies you'll benefit from nettle tea. "Nettle tea prevents hay fever and helps with allergies," said Dr. Oz. Nettle tea is effective because it contains antihistamine and anti-inflammatory compounds that help clear nasal passages. It is best to drink at least 2 cups a day during allergy season. Nettle tea is used to treat other health problems such as intestinal disorders and urinary tract infections.

Herbal teas have tremendous health benefits. Moreover, they are natural, readily available and inexpensive. Visit your local health food store and stock on on healing herbal teas.

## **Immunity Boosting Foods**

If you're tired of taking prescription drugs for common health concerns, you might want to learn about immunity boosting foods to strengthen your body's resistance to illnesses. Healthy, natural food acts as medicine in the body without causing harmful side-effects. Dr. Oz recommends the following foods based on their ability to promote positive health.

***Dark Purple and Black Grapes.*** Of all the immunity boosting food available, dark colored grapes are a leading favorite. Dark grapes are loaded with antioxidants which may help protect the body against cancer by fighting off free-radicals. Grapes are also rich in a variety of vitamins and nutrients which support overall health. Eat grapes everyday while they're in season. During off season, purchase frozen varieties. Choose organic grapes when available to reduce your intake of pesticides.

***Tahini.*** Tahini is a type of paste made from sesame seeds. It comes in roasted and natural varieties. Spread tahini on a fresh whole wheat bagel for a nutritious, filling breakfast. Tahini is rich in zinc and magnesium which boosts immunity. Tahini is believed to have anti-aging properties. It is also known to relieve constipation.

***Pumpkin.*** Another delicious immunity boosting food is pumpkin. Pumpkin is rich in beta-carotene, a powerful antioxidant. Pumpkin may help with eye problems and lessen the risk of heart disease. Pumpkin can be used to create a plethora of healthy meals and tasty desserts.

## Dr. Oz on Soda

Learn how to overcome your addiction to soda with the help of Dr. Oz. Americans spend more than $60 billion dollars a year for soda, an unhealthy product that contributes to poor health.

Soda is full of high fructose corn syrup or sugar and loaded with caffeine. Diet soda with artificial sweetener is even worse. According to Dr. Oz, soda addiction contributes to diabetes, heart disease and kidney failure.

Just like alcoholic beverages and cigarettes, the soda habit is hard to break. Dr. Oz offers 3 tips to help end the love affair with soda. First, Dr. Oz says to replace soda with orange juice. Although orange juice contains sugar, at least it provides nutrients for the body. Second, use chewing gum or soda flavored candy to help control the urge to drink soda. Dr. Oz's third tip is to drink a glass of seltzer water right before drinking soda because this will reduce the amount of soda consumed. Eventually, the desire to drink soda will be gone.

Once you overcome the soda addiction, you'll be able to focus on drinking healthy beverages. Try drinking pure water with a twist of lemon or unsweetened green tea. Drinking natural fruit juice is also a good alternative to soda. However, "It's best to dilute your juice," said Dr. Oz.

## **Foods for Memory**

If you are having trouble with your memory, try eating some of the best foods for memory recommended by Dr. Oz. Today's busy lifestyles cause many people to experience brain fog, a condition in which the mind temporarily goes blank making it impossible to remember things.

Including Dr. Oz's 6 top memory boosting foods in your diet will help you overcome lapses in memory. They are filled with essential vitamins and nutrients, delicious, affordable and available at most supermarkets.

***Rosemary.*** According to Dr. Oz, rosemary can enhance the quality of memory. Rosemary contains an antioxidant that helps protect your brain cells. So add it to your diet to enhance the flavor of your food and to boost your memory. Even the smell of rosemary is enough to stimulate your memory, so consider purchasing rosemary scented oils.

***Eggplant.*** Eggplant contains anthocyanin, a known memory boosting substance. It also contains nasunin, which is an antioxidant. "The antioxidants in eggplant protect the fat around the brain cells, " advised Dr. Oz.

***Red Onions***. Red onions also contain anthocyanin and have been used for centuries in Asia to boost memory. Dr. Oz recommends adding red onions to foods such as stir-fry dishes and sandwiches for a quick memory boost.

**Whole Wheat Noodles.** "Whole wheat noodles contain thiamine, one of the B-vitamins, which is important for building brain cells," explained Dr. Oz. Beans and nuts are also good sources of thiamine.

**Spinach.** "This leafy green vegetable is excellent for improving memory because it is rich in folic acid," said Dr. Oz. Moreover, folic acid may help protect against Alzheimer's disease. One cup of cooked spinach provides more than the daily recommended requirement of folic acid.

**Peanuts.** Peanuts are another top choice among Dr. Oz's memory boosting foods. Peanuts contain choline, which is an essential building block for the brain.

## Spices for Health

Spice up your food and improve your health with these leading herbs and spices. Dr. Oz and Dr. Joseph Mercola explained the health benefits of common spices.

*Italian Spice.* This spice is rich in antioxidants and anti-inflammatory properties.

*Thyme.* Thyme is anti-microbial and contains

antioxidants. It is often used in mouthwash.

*Sage*. Sage is beneficial for both arthritis and asthma.

*Marjoram.* Marjoram is great for digestion and as a sleep aid. It has antibacterial properties and is used as an antiseptic in some cultures.

*Oregano*. Oregano is anti-microbial and useful for fungal infections.

*Apple Pie Spice*. The ginger in apple pie spice is a natural remedy for nausea during pregnancy and seasickness.

*Jamaican Allspice*. Jamaican allspice is helpful for gas and digestion problems. It is a combination of pimento, cloves, cinnamon and nutmeg.

*Cinnamon*. Cinnamon contains anti-cancer properties and also helps lower blood sugar levels.

*Cloves*. Cloves are a rich source of antioxidants. They are known for their ability to lower blood sugar levels. In fact, cloves are more effective at reducing blood sugar than cinnamon.

***Turmeric***. Turmeric has anti-inflammatory properties and may help fight cancer.

## Conclusion

The best way to maintain and improve your health is to provide your body with high quality foods and physical activity. Learn everything you can about the benefits of natural and organic foods. Always read food labels so you can avoid products that contain known toxins. Make sure you get moderate exercise everyday and adequate sleep at night. Pay close attention to your body and how it functions so that you'll know when something is amiss. When you experience a health concern speak up in the doctor's office. Don't be afraid to ask questions and get a second opinion when necessary. In other words, take personal responsibility for your health. Start today. Tomorrow might be too late.

## *Acknowledgements*

*Thank you to the supreme being for love and guidance.*

*To my family and friends, Thank you for your love and support throughout the years.*

*To Dr. Wayne Dyer, my favorite guru, Thank you for the "Power of Intention."*

*Many thanks to Dr. Mehmet Oz for not being afraid to keep the public informed of the truth even in the face of opposition.*

## *About the Author*

*Dr. Aleathea R. Wiggins is a writer specializing in education, health and parenting. She is a former university professor, curriculum facilitator and teacher. Dr. Wiggins holds advanced degrees and credentials in journalism, education, health and childcare administration.*

Printed in Great Britain
by Amazon.co.uk, Ltd.,
Marston Gate.